COMPASSION

POWER

BEYOND

SCIENCE

MS. VICTOR BO IMANI, M.S.W., M.F.T.

ACKNOWLEDGMENT

I, Ms. Victor Bo Imani, a.k.a. Botswanna Imani hereby express my utmost gratitude to T.J. DeWitt, of the Bristol Public Library, for all his untiring support and assistance in publishing all my books.

"Compassion Power Beyond Science"

Here is Ms. Victor Bo Imani. As touched upon in the back of my books, I mention being an 'energy worker, intuitive, seer and a 'sensitive' and that I traveled to third world countries supporting others in their self-healing and initiating others to carry on the much needed support of the population in their area.

Of the very few people that I related one or another of the stories I am going to relate to you, they suggested that I share them with others. Till now, it has felt wrong. The reason for that is that these stories feel very sacred to me. They touch me deep into my core, my heart, my soul, and deeper still. I have been concerned about what some call it, "cast not pearls before swine'. I was concerned about appearing arrogant. More important, the stories instead of opening up new doors and windows for people, may, indeed, be regarded as made up fairy tales and worse, leading people on with lies and deceit. However, most importantly, I was concerned about people minimizing the stories purity, and sacredness. It is really all beyond words. You can, hopefully, somewhat feel and experience the magnanimity of the events related.

The reason I was just, today, December 7, 2019, inner guided, very clearly, to write it all down and have it go public was during a bit of news I heard this afternoon about an ophthalmologist. They stated that he restored vision to multitudes. I was intrigued. It ends up that he discovered that many people in third world countries had been regarded as blind, whereas he discovered that they only needed glasses. They further stated how valuable it is to share this information so others can also have their 'vision'.

This stirred in me, and, suddenly it felt clear it was time to share now. I am on my final journey in this life, homebound for years, and now confined to my upstairs bedroom, mostly in bed. Then besides those people whose lives were changed and those who saw or heard about it, which, in the scheme of things are a very few people. There have been many others who have been supported by what comes through me without them knowing about it. This was due to it occurring in a very different way than the stories hereby related. Why? You may wonder.

Most of the stories I am sharing below occurred in third world countries where many, still understand and accept getting well without medical intervention due to their ancestral traditional/aboriginal heritage. In the United States, however, there have only been a very small minority of people who were open and receptive to it. Therefore, the cosmos glorious energy came through me in a very different way. This was through words that came through me. Often even I was unaware of why these words, or those were said by me. I trusted that as long as I am willing and able to be a pure vessel, the best words and questions came through me to most optimally help others make a shift for their benefit. Often it made zero sense to me why this or that was said through me. Sometimes it became clear to me, later on, as to why. Often it was unnecessary for me to know. All I had to do was to trust, surrender, say and do as I was led to.

The multitudes were clueless before, during and after. Very rarely, in the United States or other Western cultured nations, became aware of the magnanimity of their occurrence after talking and or being with me. We westerners have lost so much with our scientific, realistic, educated, clever and conscious consciousness. We have lost contact with our sub-conscious which is our root selves, who we really are.

Our sub-conscious is connected to our souls, it is our foundation. It carries all our memories in our bones, muscles, and, indeed in every cell of our bodies. Our sub-conscious remembers all through time and space, including all our previous lives. Meditation, many have found, can help us reconnect with our most valuable part of our beingness, our sub-conscious. It aids us in our most important journey, as stated in the Greek mystery schools, 'know thyself'. In our sub-conscious are the treasures of 'know thyself'. Our conscious mind, regrettably, due to indoctrination, have crushed our most vital knowledge of who we really are.

Fortunate are those who are still connected to their indigenous, aboriginal ways of their ancestors. Very sadly, amongst the white people, as they made colonies, and the missionaries imposed ignorance, western mentality, has deprived the natives of their very rich heritage. With it their lost their pure, childlike openness to 'magic', to wonder, to true and heartfelt joy, love, naïvetés and purity. 'Education' has very little to say for itself. It deprives us from our most valuable inner self connection with our sub-conscious and with our soul, our spirit. Those are our most valuable commodities. Trading 'Educated minds' for really 'BEING' is a harmful and poor trade off.

Sadly, it is only a very small minority of people, once we have been indoctrinated and 'educated' who actually make it back to our true source and true selves.

Often, due to all the 'science', 'education' and greed society has chosen to value going to the moon over feeding the hungry. They value fossil fuel, nuclear weapons versus valuing nature with all its gifts. We have chosen to ignore that with each mindless action with which our air, earth, plants, trees and our environment are compromised, we are, in effect self-destructing with many diseases heretofore unknown. Some of us may yet die of the effects we have created. Others of us may be fortunate to die before we experience the full effects of our mindless behavior. In either case, we have passed this catastrophe unto future generations. We have been bad caretakers for many years of our home, Mother Earth. Beings on other planetary systems only shake their heads at our foolish, mindless, careless and cruel behaviors.

Let us, now, return to the major focus of this book. Let us all shake off the energy of the matter about our environment and shift into being open and receptive to upliftment, hope, trust, acceptance, our sub-conscious, our purity and childlike nature. Let us release our doubt, fear, and limited consciousness.

My intention is, that with each story we all hear and feel lighter and lighter. May we all hear, listen and receive that which is most beneficial for us, safely and gently.

To give you a timeline for when all this occurred:

I begin this book, in Baltimore with my job as Psychotherapist which ended about September/ October in 1994. The trip to Tanzania was in June/July of 1994. The other trips abroad were from 1994-2005. Due to a crisis/trauma event in my life I was unable to do any more traveling after 2005.

You may consider reading only one story at a time, allowing your complete mind/body/spirit to integrate, incorporate, and with that best support the shift that your beingness is ready for. You may choose to postpone reading the next story only when your inner wisdom so guides you. Or, perhaps, you may feel pulled to re-read the same story again and again, and with each re-reading hear and read it on a deeper and deeper level, benefiting more and more each and every time.

In 1992, due to several circumstances I started having memories of having been severely abused by every family member. I had already gotten involved in utilizing holistic health care years earlier. Therefore, in addition to regular 'therapies' I found a female who did 'Mariel healing' which is energy work, without touching, which is meant to support shifts. I observed what she did.

Very early on with the 'memories', I, simultaneously noticed that my hands were tingling. This was a brand new phenomenon. Having observed the female doing the energy modality I experimented with a plant. I put my hands above the leaves, several inches up from the leaves. Once the leaves followed the direction of my hands as it slowly moved back and forth, I knew that my beingness 'remembered' how to be a vessel.

Upon my first 'memories' I began twelve step meetings for addiction to relationships. Gratefully a man called Cris, after the meeting told me about a meditation center nearby. I ended up ceasing the twelve step meetings due to the pattern of people persisting in telling 'war stories'. That meant, to me, that people instead of progressing kept on recycling the yuck, and with it maintained the addictive cycle, while simultaneously, alluding themselves that they were getting weller.

Instead, I began and kept going to the meditation center. Immediately I did very well with that. I have continued to meditate since then with good results. I am very grateful.

So here I was continuing my job as a psychotherapist, and, simultaneously, focusing on my dealing with the matter of the memories.

First evidence with a client with me as a Psychotherapist.

One day an elder female came in for a session. She stated that she had heart surgery which went very well. However, the grafting of skin from her thigh that was necessary to replace skin in her heart area. That area of her thigh has been unable to heal. She was distraught because she had been used to going for a walk daily and due to the unhealed area on her thigh she was unable to go for her beloved walks.

I carefully asked her whether she would interested in trying out something very different. I dared to try this mostly as was a very open, bright, alert, and aware woman, one that I felt would be more likely to try something 'out of the box'.

 I was well aware that as a psychotherapist I was walking on questionable waters. Nevertheless, I felt it was my duty as a helper to share what I had hoped would assist the healing of the skin on her thigh. I felt and feel that when we are gifted with a skill it is meant to be shared rather than keeping it locked up.

She was open for us to try. I explained that I will put my hands several inches above the area of her wound. I further stated that she may feel heat, coolness, tingly sensation or something else. I asked her to give me feedback on what, if anything she felt. After a few seconds she stated that she felt heat from my hands going into her thigh. I then asked her to tell me when that stops or changes. After a short while she stated that the heat stopped. I was inner guided to move my hands a little further down. I again asked her to tell me what she feels. She then stated that she felt coolness from my hands. I was surprised. I was so glad that I refrained from imposing and trusted my inner wisdom to take over, otherwise how would I have known that one area needed heat and, just below that area, coolness was required. Getting out of the way, I discovered is most pertinent.

This is good wisdom both in being a vessel of energy to support another, and, indeed in all of life. Getting out of the way supports us in freeing ourselves from our conscious minds interfering with our true wisdom and discernment of our sub-conscious.

I checked in with the client. She then stated that the coolness also stopped. She thanked me and left. The next week she showed up and gleefully stated that her thigh was all healed and she was back to her daily walks. She thanked me and left.

This was my first proof that, indeed this thing works.

I then had inner guidance that, actually, I was born with this ability. However, due to all the abuse, the skill was pushed down, as if in a pressure cooker, due to the more important matter of focusing the best I could for my safety and just to stay alive. As the first memory revealed itself was when I first felt my hands tingling. As more and more memories revealed themselves, the power from my hands and heart became stronger and stronger.

Next, a mother who had come for a couple of sessions revealed that she was very concerned about her daughter aged four or five. One day her daughter's teacher noticed that the little girl who had always colored and drew pictures in the assortment of colors suddenly began coloring only with red and black. Gratefully, the teacher knew something was very wrong.

The mother took her child to a psychiatrist who found out that the little girl was sexually abused by a little boy. He gave the girl psychotropic medicine to take. The mother was concerned about her beloved child at such an early age to be taking such medication. I, was in grief. I told her we could try something and hopefully it will help. She brought in her little girl. I asked the child to lay down on the carpeted floor. I then told her that I had a vacuum cleaner in my hand, and, without asking her to relate what happened, as I knew that would be counterproductive, I explained and requested her to gently recall the harm and allow the vacuum cleaner to suck up all those memories. I was inner guided to 'vacuum' the area beneath her waist. I made vacuuming humming sounds and make circles with my vacuum cleaner around her stomach until I was inner guided that it was done.

Of course I wanted to know the results. I had prepared a blank paper and a box of crayons. The important thing was what colors would she select? Gratefully, instead of only red and black, which indicated rage, anger and deep woundedness, the beloved child picked up and drew with yellows, pinks, blues and other bright colors with a smile on her face.

Her mother returned to state that her child was taken off the psychotropic drugs and that her teacher reported that her little girl was back to herself as she was before the trauma.

That was two for two.

Next a mother came in for a session and expressed her great distress about her teenage daughter. The mother related that her daughter was a very diligent student, a very well behaved child and suddenly, she started to hear voices telling her to kill herself. A psychiatrist gave her psychotropic drugs. With that her beloved child became a zombie. I dared, yet again, to offer an alternative solution that, hopefully, would help. The mother was interested. She had, previously told me of her deep religious beliefs also shared by her daughter. I asked for clear inner guidance.

When the mother and daughter showed up for the session I explained that what was called for was an 'exorcism' of this being who was telling her daughter to kill herself. Her daughter being of pure heart and spirit with a gentle nature was an easy target for an energy intent on being a parasite off her. I requested both mother and daughter to pray in their way, and that I will do the same.

Fortunately, there was a door to the outside grassy area next to where we were sitting. I was inner guided to open the door to best facilitate the yuckeed energy to leave. I was inner guided to demand the harmful energy to leave, first to myself, and then out loud. The two, mother and daughter prayed their way as I continued to powerfully demand the being to leave and never return. Finally felt it leave. Of course I was without any knowledge of whether it left for good or would return.

 Several weeks later the mother returned with great news. The messages to the daughter directing her to kill herself never returned since our session. The psychiatrist took the daughter off the drugs. Similarly, like with the little girl, the teenager returned to her gentle self. She reverted back to doing very well with her schoolwork as well as helping her mother with house chores as she always did beforehand.

That was three for three.

Next, a family came in. a couple, their son about age nine or ten and a daughter who was a teen-ager. I noticed immediately that the girl was dressed all in black. It felt off for me. The mother and two children expressed upsetness at their father was so pent up that his leg always shook and his constant pent up way of being was very difficult and stressful for them all.

I, yet again, offered to try something different with the father. Upon their consent I asked the children to go out into the waiting room. I requested that the husband move off the sofa he was sitting on and, instead sit in a chair. I was inner guided to direct energy over his head. Suddenly his complete body started shaking as if he was having an epileptic seizure. I became quiet frightened, however, since I was clearly guided to continue, I did. I was actually, quiet surprised and relieved that the wife said nothing. It appears that she, for some reason trusted what was happening. After more shaking, it finally stopped and the father sat still on the chair. At our next meeting the family reported that the father had become calm and stayed so, and how relieved they all were at his steadiness and calm demeanor.

Then the parents and brother brought up the issue of the teenager always wearing black and that they were very concerned about it. They had gone to the pediatrician however he made zero recommendations. With the son sent out of the room, again, I requested the girl to sit in a chair, and again I was inner guided to put my hands over her head and focus on the energy to flow through me into her.

Well, at our next meeting, the girl was a changed woman. She wore an outfit in two shades of blue and she was smiling. The family shared that the daughter had left her previous friends who all wore black and now had new friends that she hung out with. The family was most happy.

That was five for five.

However, a short while later, the director of the center called me in and stated that a pediatrician called her up and related the matter of the teen-age girl getting well. He complained that it was inappropriate for a psychotherapist to do what I did. Apparently, the family who had told him again and again about their concern for their daughter and he never did anything to help her, related to him about her recovery and how it occurred. He, however, instead of being thrilled and happy that finally the teen-ager was well, chose, instead to go into the darkness of jealousy.

He also chose to eliminate his rival, me, by doing his best to eliminate any future interference, an 'interference' that he perceived was made to make him look bad and incompetent. The truth was, he never even made any suggestions to possible solutions to the matter and totally disregarded their concerns.

I would hope he felt some shame and guilt, however my inner guidance states to me otherwise. He was a self-centered ego-maniac who had zero business being a physician, much less a pediatrician.

Therefore, the manager gave me an ultimatum that I either refrain from doing such activity in the future or leave.

I was aware, from the first, before offering support to the clients in a 'different way' of the importance of refraining from physically touching clients. Gratefully, the energy that came through me was without any need to touch. It felt right for me both regarding the others that would be receptive and also for me. Due to my 'stories' I felt uncomfortable with touching others. The energy was such that I discovered that it could be sent across the room, across the country, and indeed, anywhere at all and be most effective. Intention was all it needed. You may wonder how do I know this, or did I just assume that it worked. Well, I had confirmation and validation time and time again from people I actually had communication with on the telephone and/ or face to face.

And, yes, there can be a great value at closeness between the recipient and I. This, being: the placement of my hands a few inches above their body. There is also the importance of having options. First, how much 'closeness' does the other and I feel comfortable with. It is important to gage that, each time and with each client and to choose the most optimum distance accordingly. Do we need/prefer being across the room from each other? Would the preference rather be setting up a time, when they are at their home, when the energy was to be sent? Or was it best to send it along without them knowing when? Options are best instead of the client feeling boxed in and with that making the success of the matter being compromised or even being counterproductive.

I was also aware that utilizing this or any other different modality to support was lacking in the 'job description' of a psychotherapist. And, since I was inner guided to 'utilize' the skill I was just made aware of, I felt obliged to do so.

 Inner guidance, a new awareness that came with meditation was my most valuable commodity that I cherished and continue deeply valuing in my life. I am most grateful. Our unique skills, gifts or whatever we wish to call it, are meant to be shared. That is why we have them. The same as sharing information which can offer others alternate options available to them which they were unaware of, beforehand. My great motto of 'power to the people', is a banner I have carried for eons and I enjoy waving it around.

The ultimatum given was an easy one to reply to for me. I was gifted with this ability at birth. It has been restored as the memories freed the energy that allowed this wonder to come through me. It was clear to me that my path is to be a care giver, to support others in their journey into health and wellbeing. I was now aware of two different ways to best facilitate my task. This being both as a psychotherapist and an energy worker. We are meant to share our gifts to benefit others and the world to be a safer, more peaceful and healthier home for all.

I left my job.

Previous to this ultimatum, I had been inner guided to go to Tanzania to do research on 'Epic folklore and fable' run by Greenpeace. It was a two week project. I made arrangements to stay in Tanzania for four weeks, allowing two weeks with the Greenpeace group and two weeks by myself, following the directives I was being given in bits and pieces while I was still in America.

I remember, upon my return from Tanzania, several members of the staff remarked how I had changed from before my trip abroad. This, absolutely was very clear to me also.

Once I decided to go on the trip, I made arrangements with Greenpeace, the airplane, and with the company I worked for. I began getting more and more information on the upcoming journey to West Africa. By that time, my meditations had become more refined, and with it, more beneficial.

You may wonder how the trip to Tanzania came about.

First, I would like to state that contrary to many professionals, my outlook was to have people for as few sessions as possible. 'Get done what needs to be and get on with your life on your own'. That was my way. I stayed away from catering to dependency. The sessions described in the above stories were the only sessions those people had with me. With strong inner guidance, we immediately focused on the root of the matter, got it done and they went on their way. Typically, the client choose how often and when they wished to return. One caveat on this were clients that were mandated by the court system to have a certain amount of sessions. Even then we stayed focused on their independence, their self-sufficiency to best facilitate the prevention of them needing to be 'mandated' by the courts again.

Now I will relate as to how the trip to Tanzania came about. One of my clients, in session, somehow, for some reason, I am unable to recall how it came about, told me about Greenpeace and their wonderful work in and around the world. As he related they invite individuals to join them in their assortment of projects for a two week period in which a Greenpeace staff heads and, for the Tanzania project, for example, local college students also participated. Besides the air fare, there was a charge for lodging and for the privilege of being part of the adventure. I asked the client whether he had some more information. He stated that, as a matter of fact he gets regular mailings from them regarding upcoming projects. I asked him whether he can bring it to me to read. This he did. At home before opening up the catalogue I requested my inner guidance that if I am meant to go to any of the projects that were in many parts of the world, for me to be clearly led to which one.

I slowly and mindfully looked through the most interesting catalogue. There was this project in Europe, that project hither and others yonder. Each had a picture and the description. Suddenly, there it was. My heart started shifting very perceptibly. This was it, the project in Tanzania. In Tanzania, like in most indigenous countries, forever stories were told. There was a very rich culture of Epic Folklore and Fable in Tanzania. However, they had never been written down. Awareness came of the importance of writing them down for posterity. To keep the culture, the ancient valuable stories needed to stay alive. With time and changes, there was the increased danger of the stories being lost. The projects job was to write down these stories and give them to schools, libraries and other places that would keep them safe. They were to be archived. I felt this was most important for us all. Treasures beyond compare.

Globally speaking, there have always been stories passed down from generation to generation. The elders, the wise ones carried and told them. Stories have this wonderful power that shares and relates wisdoms and knowledge in a way that expands others awareness in an easy and palatable way. Where regular 'teaching' could and would fail, stories succeeded. People let their guard down, perked up and listened with their heart and soul. The conscious mind out of the way, the inner child comes forth to play and ends up learning. The same story can be heard again and again and, each time there is a new and expanded understanding. Our circumstances change and with it we change. Therefore, our attention can be drawn to aspects of the story we were unable to hear on previous occasions. With our inner scenery changes comes our outer scenery doing the same. It is quiet fascinating.

On the photo included with the write up about the project in Tanzania, was a photo of a few tribal people.

Then I had two very intense meditations. In the first one I felt myself surrounded by some Massai tribal members. They identified themselves as Massai tribal members and stated: 'come, we need you.' I wish to clarify that the Greenpeace project had nothing to do with the Massai. For the project I had to go to a place called Mwanza, close to the center of Tanzania. Through research I found out that the Massai tribe resided mostly in Kenya, however there were also some in the Northern part of Tanzania called Arusha. My plan was that after the two weeks with Greenpeace I would travel to Arusha to be with the people who called me to come to them.

There was a requirement by Tanzania, due to a great epidemic of Malaria, that all visitors get inoculated to prevent one from getting malaria. For those that are unaware, the malaria virus is contracted by being bit by a malaria carrier insect, the mosquito. I was very afraid. I spoke to the homeopathic physician I was going to. I had left the regular medical field to avoid their intrusive and invasive ways that I had found to be very damaging to me. The Homeopathic physician suggested that I refrain from getting the vaccine as it was harmful to my system and that the dangers of the vaccine outweighed the chances of contracting malaria. I was afraid.

Then I had my second major meditation. I suddenly felt that inside me was a lion. I felt its tail under me. I felt its mane around my head. He identified himself as a lion from Tanzania. He stated, 'we the lions await your coming to Tanzania. You will be safe from the big animals, the lions and tigers and from the tiny animals, the mosquitoes. We greet you and look forward to your coming.' I cried and cried, quiet overwhelmed. In effect the lion reassured me that I was going to be safe without getting the vaccine. The fear left me.

Interestingly, the only time the issue of avoiding getting the vaccine only came up when I went to Zanzibar, part of Tanzania and yet somewhat separate. After my plane landed I had to go through custom inspection and the officer saw in my documents that I had never received the vaccine. He stated that I had to get the vaccine or I was unable to enter. I am unsure how I got the courage and the strength to say to him boldly, that I would leave Zanzibar rather than get the vaccine. He saw and felt that I meant it. I am without any memory if he discussed it with another officer or if he made the decision by himself all I know is he allowed me to enter. I was and am aware that the main reason for him allowing me in anyway was a monetary one. Zanzibar would lose the income I would spend in my time there. There could also have been the fear of me making a fuss which could have kept other foreign visitors from going to Zanzibar. Again a money thing, and bad publicity. He chose wisely. I stayed. More on Zanzibar later.

The project was slated to begin in June. I signed up for the first two weeks. Upon my arrival I found out that I was the only 'outsider'. There was, of course, the staff member from Greenpeace who was from the States. Then there were the college students of the Dar Es Salaam University and the two leaders for them and whoever joined the project. This made for my two weeks much different than had there been more 'outsiders'. I, in effect, was taken to native 'medicine woman and men', invited to stay at one of their homes and other attention I could have never gotten had there been more attendees.

At our first group meeting, there was discussion of who was going to do what. Then it was my turn. I, shyly shared that there is this energy that comes through me that supports others in their healing. They designated me as the 'healer'. I have learned that the term 'healer' is, actually off. I believe, given beneficial circumstances, people actually 'heal themselves'. I believe 'dis-ease' in ones beingness, be it mind, body or spirit occurs, mainly from lack of feeling lovable, loved. This also include having low self-esteem, feeling undeserving and related matters. With this the immune system is compromised and the being gets unwell, with the most vulnerable areas being the first to be effected. People respond well when they feel accepted, sincerely cared for, respected, loved and truly listened to. This, gratefully, comes through me and what some would call 'magic' occurs. Voila!

The first example came up, best I recall, was when we went to a small group of village people. I am unable to remember much of that incident except for this one female having some challenges which got tended to through me and the matter vanished. For some reason she totally ignored me. She talked and visited with the staff of Greenpeace. To date I feel bad about that. Regardless of my clearly evolving, my ego still feels bad, totally ignored and, indeed disregarded totally by the one who benefited from the energy which was only effective due to my true caring. I hope in the future I will be healthy enough to be free from needing or desiring that validation. I feel petty. Obviously, there is always more growth to be done, regardless of what level we may have achieved in any area. For me it was the feeling of 'what about me? How come you are totally disregarding me as if I was without even existing?' Thank you, dear reader, for hearing my limited consciousness regarding this matter that still feels bad after so many years.

The next opportunity for my 'job' presented itself when I went to stay at one of the students' home. I was given a bed to sleep on in the room where their very beautiful daughter slept. In the evening, the woman of the house, wife of the student, mother of the girl, told me she had gotten malaria from a mosquito bite. She described how it was affecting her and I proceeded in being a vessel on her behalf. She immediately, like the others, felt a shift and a release. She was grateful.

The next opportunities presented themselves, ironically, when different students offered to take me to Medicine women and men. First they took me to a Female medicine woman, she practiced in her indigenous heritage ways. However, when we arrived she was unwell. She stated that she had eaten the flesh of an 'old goat' and it made her ill. I offered to support her. This she consented to and, sure enough she got well. Then it was my turn, as she was feeling well. She called upon a few of her people, and we all went into a tent. I was instructed to lay down, had a big white cloth covering me at about a two feet distance above my body, just enough so I only saw the sheet and I never saw those who were in the tent with me, the drummers. Several of them began to drum.

I love the sound of drums. I have found drumming resonates very strongly and beneficially with me. First of all I have a tendency to have challenges being 'present'. The sound of drums, especially when it is close and personal as it was in that little tent that afternoon. The drumming resounded in my complete beingness.

As a matter of fact, in many traditions drums have been utilized in assisting people in making shifts in their total mind/body and spirit wellness and being 'transported' into expanded consciousness.

The truth of the matter was, however, in this instance, as much as I liked it, it lacked some major ingredients, therefore very much limiting the value that it would have otherwise been. Perhaps they were just going through the motions rather than truly being in or with it?

Next I was taken to another native medicine being, a male. I was taken up the mountain to where he was by a young man with major physical challenges. He spoke enough English that I offered to him, if he so chose, to receive energy that could possibly support him. He responded with uproarious laughter. That meant no. I felt, and others confirmed, that he was perfectly content, and even happy with his condition. This was because his condition freed him from having to work or fend for himself as his complete community took care of his every need. Why upset and ruin what was, for him, perfect. There it was. I offered, I did my share, as good as if more had happened.

The medicine man greeted me in a tent. All Tanzanians have dark skin. Some a little lighter others darker. This medicine man, a handsome, robust man's skin was jet black, his pearly white teeth glistened against his glorious face. He was dressed all in black. His energy was huge and fantastic. I could have stared at him all day long without detracting from my amazement at his energy and looks. He did his work by shaking around some bones in a container and then pouring them on the carpet we both sat on. He stated some findings.

On the site we were on, actually, was his hospital. There were tents all around for his 'patients' to have their own space to heal. It appeared that he also lived in his hospital. Before the young man took me back down the mountain a photograph was taken with the two men with enormous smiles. I kept the photograph for many years. Each time, I looked at it I fondly remembered and smiled. And each time I wished I could be with that medicine man again, just to be in his and with his amazing energy. WOW! What a gift to us all. I can, actually as I write this, feel nostalgia and feel his energy with me. Ahhh, if only in the flesh. However, perhaps this way is even better.

The next medicine man to be taken to was one who combined his native ways and his christian education. He was a male short of stature and very thin. We both sat on the ground, in his home in a small room. He had a bowl of water in front of him. He donned a red headdress and kept on looking into the water to get information. He, then, shared it with me. What he stated resonated with me, though it was nothing of great significance, as I recall.

What I do clearly recall, was how noticeably he got very tired after the 'reading'. Upon my questioning him, he stated that he always gets very tired after a reading. I offered to be a vessel and he eagerly accepted. He was revived instantly. Some wisdoms were shared with him on how he may best proceed on his own in the future to prevent his being so depleted. We talked some more and we exchanged mailing addresses he walked me to public transportation and we both felt a strong kinship with each other. I sent him a mailing and he sent me a post card with some kind words, and, again expressing his gratitude.

The next visit to two other medicine men was yuckee and therefore I will refrain from saying more. The reason I am saying this amount is just to share that it is soooo important to have the wisdom and discernment, regardless of who the other is. What do they really stand for and with? Or who they say they are and who claim they are two opposites? Instead of giving and supporting are they really vampires, stealing energy from others for their own behalf, and charging for it to boot. A double whammy. It took quite a while to free myself from the yuck of that visit. I hope I am totally free of that toxicity and all directly and indirectly related to it and them.

Then on to two young men who worked together utilizing the Muslim medicine path. They opened up the Koran to give them the answers. Without me sharing any information, they stated that they were informed that healing comes through me in two different ways. Quite amazing, I said to myself. I then shared that I am a practicing psychotherapist and another way.

Well, they were interested in the 'other' way. For the first time, and later in my journeys I was directed time and time again to do something new. I was inner guided to initiate these two young men with the ability to be a vessel of energy to support others in their healing in yet, another beneficial way. This, in effect was the baton being passed to them, and, simultaneously, me still having the skills on my own.

Perhaps passing the baton is confusing. Perhaps giving them their own baton may be a better way to phrase it. Or maybe cloning a duplicate or a baton specially formed for their and their clients' needs would be even better. In either case, I like the term 'passing the baton' and, therefore that is how I will continue stating it this way from here on in with these writings. Thank you for remembering for the next times I use that term.

They were most grateful for that. I hope they have used it wisely. The quieter one of the two requested to speak to me alone. We did so outside. I was then inner guided to tell him that what I was getting was for him to do work on his own so that he may truly 'come into his own', instead of being a backdrop to the other. He expressed his relief at hearing this. He further stated that he had thought about this very same idea, but was unsure of which way to go with it. He was most grateful and stated that he would now make his own way.

I hope he did so and has succeeded, his heart energy was extraordinary. It is the compassionate heart that really makes the difference. The head and power energy is one thing, however, the heart energy, ah yes, that is the stuff that true and fruitful shifts are made of.

The final medicine man story that comes to mind at this time was my visit to a medicine man who combined the native way and the Muslim traditions. When I first arrived I was directed to an empty room to sit and wait in. Later, I was led into where the medicine was awaiting me. He had very dignified and vibrant energy. He wore a bright shiny blue cloak that had long billowy sleeves. Indeed it was billowy altogether. It was without any zippers, buttons or any fastenings. It appeared to me that he had to done it over his head. As you may notice, I was quiet fascinated by his attire. It spoke to who and what he stood for. It all resonated.

He stated that he was informed, like the two young had, that healing comes through me in two different ways.

Then he proceeded with putting some herbs in a large bowl of water, put it on the floor and directed me to put my feet in there. Then he wrote up some Muslim verses on a piece of paper and put it into the water with the herbs.

After the ceremony he invited me to have lunch with him. During eating he related to me that a distraught mother had brought her infant baby over. He discovered that the baby had been infected with cerebral malaria. He did whatever he could, however the infant made zero improvement. The medicine man asked whether I would be willing to see what could come through me to help. I replied in the affirmative, and stated, I would do my best.

 A while later, the mother and baby showed up. We were led downstairs, into a basement area, which was empty. I did the usual, opening up myself to be a pure and clear vessel to assist and support the infant into wellness. Typically, when I did so, it came through me gently and softly and then on to the client. This time, however it was very different. The energy came into me very powerfully, so much so that I had to allow my physical body to vibrate very quickly to prevent my body from exploding. I grabbed a hold of a post right next to me to prevent me from falling over.

 Finally, it softened and then stopped. I opened my eyes and saw the mother smiling at me broadly as her baby was cooing and moving its arms. All was well.

I was overwhelmed at all this. I stayed outside for a while in the spot where I ha soaked my feet in the water, the paper with the verses on it and the herbs. It was a lovely area. It had a round metal table with four chairs around it. Overhead there was covering made of wood criss crossing with a vine almost covering it completely. It was a great place, a pleasant, peaceful spot, with shade for me to just sit and to take in all that had just occurred. I stayed a while and then I left.

Truly an event to remember. After this, I had other occasions when the energy came through very strongly, when that amount was needed for the shift. I was more prepared then.

The final female medicine being utilized the Muslim traditions. For the journey to the Muslim female medicine woman two students of my group with the Greenpeace project actually came with and stayed with me the complete time. It was the only time any of the group stayed with me. They came to translate and support me. They were a female called Aisha and a male called Mohamed. Both were Muslim.

We climbed up the steep mountain to the healers place. We went inside the tent and waited and waited. Finally she came out and apologized for the delay. She explained that she had gotten all ready, she thought, and in the last minute she was guided to change her garment, which she proceeded to do. She was dressed all in white, a big drippy cloth also covering her head. Only her face and hands showed. She sat down and opened her Koran.

She then proceeded to allow sounds to come forth from her throat and belly. I was unsure what I meant. Then, she in the Arabic language proceeded to talk. Aisha and Mohamed translated: "We, the lions, welcome you to Tanzania. You will be safe from the big animals, the lions and tigers and the small ones including the mosquitoes. Thank you for coming to us". This was almost verbatim what I heard in my meditation in America. I understood that the sounds that came out from the woman's belly and throat were lion roars. I sobbed and sobbed. Verbatim almost the same words I was told.

And here was a medicine woman on the other side of the world, from the northern to the southern hemisphere, with totally opposite energy from one another, even water flows down the drain in the opposite circle direction. Even so she was repeating the message I received from the lions, here in her tent. It was, as you may possibly imagine, beyond hu-being comprehension. Definitely very un-scientific!

Then the meeting was done. The medicine woman accompanied us out. Typically, she stated, she only accompanies visitors to the outside of her tent. However, she stated, that she was so touched by our meeting that she actually accompanied us half-way down the mountain. There we were walking together, the four of us, in silence walking down from her mountain top. It was a great transition, soft and sweet from the awesome visit back into the world. I felt much supported by the three escorts. In that moment in time, contrary to my usual way of feeling, I felt that I had a loving and caring family after all.

Was that an amazing story or what?!

Getting back to earth and my Greenpeace group.

We went to various events in the community related to the project at hand. One such was going to a ceremony to initiate a new Medicine man. There had been a private ceremony attended by specific elders who had the wisdom and power to the necessary steps to make this happen. And, in addition, there was the ceremony my team and others were welcome to attend. Before the ceremony began, the medicine man to be, who, apparently had been told about me requested that I support in having the pain in his leg in its healing. This done, a female approached and stated that she has been unable to get pregnant. Again, I opened myself up to be a vessel on her behalf. Years later I was informed that she had given birth to three healthy children and all was well.

At the ceremony there were females who danced around in a circle, nothing showy, just walking around to the rhythm of some gentle music. I am unable to recall whether it was chanting or some instrument, however I do specifically joining in the dancing.

 Then there was what was very upsetting to me, the sacrifice of a lamb. Though it was done out of my view, however, hearing the lamb bleating deeply disturbed me.

Then I recall the new medicine man posing this way and that. An elder put some herb on the new medicine man's tongue. There were piles of bags, apparently with paraphernalia associated with his new title. The bags were off to the side, leaning on a building door in full view. All of this was a powerful experience for me.

Another event we went to was a singing contest. There was the group the leaders of my team were affiliated with and another group. The event began with the two contestants taking turn in chanting and singing. I was unable to understand some of its rhyme or reason or its progress.

However, at some point there was a man in the center of the circle, by himself, and felt myself propelled to join him. He shifted his weight this way and that. I, instinctively moved my legs and shifted my weight this way and that. Suddenly there was incredible clapping and one of the leaders of my team informed me that his group had just won the contest. He further stated that this was due to me entering the circle and moving this way and that.

It appears that whatever movements my body made exhibited superiority over the other contestant. He told me that he had taken photos of the event. Later, to his chagrin later in the evening he found that his camera and film with the photos on it had been stolen. He stated that, apparently he was off in taking the photos as it was too sacred and pure to be recorded on camera. He then gifted me with the name his mother was called. This was his way to honor my contribution to the contest.

As stated I was totally a vessel and absolutely unaware of what and why. When one is a truly vessel it is almost like being a puppet with the cosmos pulling the strings. As long as what occurs is in harmony with honoring, respect and to benefit all that is true and fair, I am game. It is vital to always have clear intention, and, hopefully to be aware and to be inner guided as to when the puppeteer is from a source other than beneficial and to refrain from allowing it to take over. Mindfulness and discernment are vital!

On another occasion, we went to, yet another ceremony where there were fables recited. In the beginning, a man with a very long instrument had it 'sing'. It was quiet lovely. Then the one who was the main 'performer' the one to recite fables invited me and another of the team to lunch. We sat in a tent, on the floor and I recall a big bowl of a grain being placed in the center of the low table we sat around. Both men dug in with their fingers, scooped up grain and placed it into their mouths. I did my best to do the same, never had done this before. I barely succeeded. My self-consciousness took over. Although looking back, I doubt they would have cared this way or that. I guess I was afraid of them laughing at me for dropping the food before it got to my mouth.

One day, as the two weeks were coming to a close, one of the young men of my team approached me and stated that he has been preparing himself to partake in a marathon walk, however his ankle had developed pain and he was unable to practice. He really wanted to participate and could I help? I had him sit in a chair and was about to direct energy by his ankle when I was clearly inner guided to direct the energy on his head. I was surprised, however I did as I was told. After a bit I was inner guided that it was done. Weeks after my return to the states I received a post card from the young man that his ankle had gotten well and he was able to participate in the marathon. He was most happy and grateful.

I was taken by the team to a native medicine man, who, actually was talked about as a Doctor, to meet him and have a chat. We talked for a while. Then he asked me whether I would be willing to see if I could assist with some difficult cases that he was unable to help with. I replied yes. The group arrived. One female had lost her voice, another was covered with a rash over her entire body, and a third had some aches and pains. All got well immediately, as usual. We talked again and he kept calling me Doctor. Apparently in Tanzania, and with many indigenous/ aboriginal people they regard anyone who, like me, is able to support and help in others getting well, without getting a 'medical degree in medical school' is considered to be a doctor. I can definitely identify with that.

Before I left he asked if I would consider one more client of his. Upon hearing my affirmative he took me over to a teen age boy, on whom, he explained he had done surgery on his mouth due to a growth. The surgery went well, he stated, however the mouth was unable to heal. Well, a vessel I became and I went back to my team where we were all located.

 The next day my team and I all went on some other adventure to hear and listen to more fables. Upon our return I was informed that the doctor of the day before, who had requested from me to help with the, teen age boys mouth came to tell me that the boys' mouth was all healed. Now please remember, hardly anyone had a telephone. The way from where he was to where my team was located was without public transportation. Therefore the doctor walked two hours each way to inform me of the boys' mouth having completely healed. Quite incredible! I was disappointed that he and I missed each other. I am very grateful that he made the long trip to share the good news. I hope I told the group to express to him my gratitude for his consideration and thoughtfulness in 'walking the extra miles'. Extraordinary man, his clients and community was/is fortunate to have him. I wish him well.

That was the end of my two weeks with the Greenpeace project. I left Mwanza and went to take a bus to my next destination, Arusha to visit with the Massai tribe. That was the plan. I got to the bus station, located the bus to Arusha and looked to find the usual luggage department on the side of buses. Well, there was none. Then I saw a man, who was the driver, take luggage from people, and be it suitcases, large bags, cages with fowl in it and other baggage that I could easily see that would have been too heavy for a horse to lift. And here was the tiny man putting the items on his shoulder, climbing on a ladder, carrying the baggage and organizing the items on the roof of the bus. My heart went out to him.

 Eventually we were on our way. To get any air one could only open a window that was the only option. Gratefully I got a window seat. This afforded me the option of opening it up AND, maybe more importantly gave me a view to see and experience. We were going to pass by the edge of the Ngorongoro National Park that housed a large variety of animals. As the bus was passing the park I saw herds of antelope, giraffe, zebras and a variety of birds. Mostly many antelope and similar in that family. I ohhd and ahhd and gasped. I was and am so grateful to have seen them in their native habitat, free to roam in safety. What a treat. The best I could tell I was the only one on the bus that day to really enjoy seeing them, the rest of the people on the bus were natives for whom, probably the view was familiar. They may have gotten to the place of taking it for granted? Finally we arrived.

I went to a small establishment for my stay close to where I had been informed Massai lived in their own enclave. When I went to wash up and gazed into the mirror I was surprised to see my face looked beige and yellow from a deep layer of dust that had made themselves at home on my face. Oh, yes, the gift of having the window next to me that I opened for air, and with it also received a very thick layer of dust glued on to my face. A lot of scrubbing was needed.

The next day I seeked out and found the cultural officer who was a delegate to the Massai. I requested an opportunity to visit with the Massai. He informed me that outsiders were forbidden into their closed community and if I desired to see them, I needed to go to a hotel where they perform their 'dancing' and singing' in their native clothing. I insisted that this was contrary to why I came. Upon getting refused, I first explained that I came to the country at the request of the Massai. I also shared that I come with a gift for the Massai people. Upon his questioning, I described what it was.

Upon this he somehow contacted one of the Massai group leaders and arranged for a meeting with him.

Again please remember, mostly, contact had to be made via walking by oneself or sending messages from one to the next, to the next being, down the line to its final destination. There was very little local public transportation, mostly just buses taking people to far places, like the bus I took from Mwanza to Arusha, hours away, non-stop. Please also remember I was, during my entire time in Tanzania in very small towns, villages, or in the mountains. Many had to walk miles just to get water. I never saw anyone have a car of their own. Good roads were also in non-existence. This is how it is in a very large parts of the world.

I am just reminded, while still in Mwanza, some village people begged me to stay with them forever. They stated that will they build me a home of my own, take care of me, if only I would be there for them, for their health and wellbeing. They also stated that other villagers and communities wish the same.

I, too, wished I could stay. The Tanzanian people felt good to be with. Africa called to me very strongly in my heart. I remembered all of our true ancestors. All of peoplehood began in Africa 4.4 million years ago. Our ancestress was 'Ardi'. Her fossil remnants were found in Ethiopia fairly recently. Previously it was thought that 'Luci', who's fossil was located in the same general area of the 'Ardi' fossil years earlier was thought to be our ancestress. Years had passed since then, and with it deeper layers of the earth were revealed, dating back to earlier times. After archeologists 'found' Ardi, they carefully, for years examined her remains. They discovered that due to the differences of the bone structures of Luci and Ardi, Ardi was definitely our ancestress due to her bone structure being in alignment with ours. The lineage of Luci became extinct.

We all began in Africa, we were all dark brown or black skinned. It was only much later that we people from Africa ventured out and, eventually, relocated ourselves in various parts of Mother Earth. Due to different climates, amounts of sun exposure, availability of food and multiple variables, some of us became either very white skinned, various shades of beige, brown, red, and yellow. Some of us got blond hair, red, brown and black. We got different shapes and color of eyes, different heights and body structure. Really all of this is quite fascinating! Then different languages, life styles, different foods evolved. These different variables developed to the environment weather and what was available due to the land formations, how close or far the ocean was and so forth.

 A study found that our skin, for those readers of this book whose skin is presently white, that our skin color turned from black to white very quickly, in the scheme of things. Only a few thousand years. Quiet interesting!

I knew none of this before my trip to Tanzania. I only found all this out around five years ago, while doing some research. What I did realize, back in 1994, was that when my feet first touched Tanzanian soil that 'I Had Come Home, Home to Africa'. My skin was black just fairly recently.

Therefore the invitation by the people of that village, and people of the surrounding areas, promising to take care of me, that they wish me to stay with them, was very inviting. Very sadly, upon being with it again and again I had to recognize and admit to myself that I was too limited, too scared.

 I was born in Budapest, the capital of Hungary. We then moved to New York City, in the United States. I, later moved to Philadelphia, and then to Baltimore. In all three of those places I either lived in the 'inner cities', or adjacent to them. The inner city means that I lived in the area that was multicultural with peoples of different races, religions living together. Most of the people were of the lower income category or slightly more. The reason I am mentioning this is to clarify that I lived in a more humble way than peoples with more income. Therefore, by being 'afraid' had nothing to with expecting or desiring 'too much'.

Of course, it is all a matter of whose perspective and expectations we are referring to. The level of living I experienced in both Hungary and the United States, both being 'developed' countries, were by its very term and definition identifies them to be very different than in a third world countries, for example, like Tanzania. Therefore their standard of living and mine were very different. I am aware that there are those people, in the United States who are very used to camping out for days or longer, out in nature, without having water, toilets and so forth and be happy with it. How many of those people would be willing to live like that forever? I am also aware that there are those people like me who move to underdeveloped countries and stay there? From those people that I know of who did that, they lived in the big cities, where they actually had their basic needs covered.

If I did move to Tanzania, living in Dar Es Salaam, the capital of Tanzania in 1994, held and holds zero interest. The only places I would want to live was where I was invited. Living with the village people, in the mountains, or just out away from any big city. I craved and longed to live in nature. I wished to live and be in places that I was in during my time in Tanzania.

And, yes, I, the female staff of Greenpeace, and the two leaders had accommodations with toilets, running water, electricity, a bed to sleep in. The structure was a building rather than a tent or some other makeshift one. The students of the University remained living in their own homes. The Mwanza area which is where we were was located close enough for them to come to our meeting place and from there we, together went to our destination of the day.

 However, the people lacked all that. I was being invited to live like them. And that is what I wished I could do.

At this time I wish to as an interesting tell you about two very interesting cultural differences. The first that I was fascinated by was when I complimented a team member on something they had. I forget if it was an article of clothing or what it was. What I VERY clearly recall is that they offered it to me. I, respectfully declined and expressed my utmost gratitude. One of the two leaders explained to me that this was part of their culture. As he stated it:, "if I have two shirts and you compliment the one I am wearing, I will give you the shirt I am wearing, after all, I only need one shirt". Quite amazing! From then on in I avoided complimenting anyone in Tanzania.

The second I wish to share was. Presumably we had a schedule. Let us say the leaders stated that the next morning we were to meet at ten in the morning. I arrived on time. The female staff and two leaders arrived on time. The students varied. Some came sometimes on time, sometimes a little later, sometimes much later, or not at all. There was zero phones. Therefore none could call to explain this or that. Typically the leaders decided, each day, as to how long we all would wait before leaving for our adventure of the day.

I recall one specific day in which we waited VERY long, till the leaders decided for us to head on anyway. The next day we found out what had occurred. This is what he told us: He left his home to come and meet us. On his way, his father-in-law who noticed him walking by called to him to come in and visit. He did so. As he stated, "it was impossible for him to refuse the invitation". Everyone in the group except me, and perhaps the staff member from Greenpeace, a girl from the U.S. understood. I thought to myself: Quite Extraordinary! Cultural differences.

 It is vital to be aware that there are small or very large variables in what is expected, appropriate in one culture and yet is totally the opposite in another, and to respect it. I was a guest in Tanzania, this was their home. Humility, honoring and respecting was an absolute basic necessity.

Returning to my grappling with the invitation from the villagers. I recognized and I admitted to myself that I totally lacked all skills to suddenly move to an area where there were so many hardships I never had to deal with. The big cities were and are very short of a utopia. Many hardships existed, especially in the inner cities where I mostly lived. However the hardships were very different. We had hot and cold running water, electricity to give us light in the darkness, heat in the cold, and some of us air conditioning units for the heat. We had telephones. In the big cities where I lived, there was plenty of public transportation, as the masses, my family included, were without cars. There were stores walking distance away for us to purchase produce and other foods. As you read, the list can go on and on.

All these things, even the very basic of availability of water to drink and food to eat took great effort to get in Tanzania in the area I was invited to move to. I was especially painfully aware of the need of **me having to walk miles to get water**, screamed out to me. We could live without food for quite a while, without water we die very quickly. Every part of our beingness, even our skin craves water. Please remember, 75% of our physical body is made up of water.

Very sadly, I knew I lacked the skills, the knowledge, the strength and courage to even begin to make such a commitment. To date I grieve. I wish I could have and would have. If only I could have returned to where I began, in Africa. Alas, no. I lament and sorrow at my limitations.

The cultural officer and I arrived at the edge of the Massai village where, it was arranged I would meet with a representative of the village. I, again, stated my request and offered the gift. He called in several elders to come to our meeting. Again I related my offer and request. They laughed, apparently totally unfamiliar with such a phenomenon. Then one put out his leg that was hurting him and, in effect stated, 'show me'. Well in seconds he was convinced. I was afforded access to their community.

 The next day, the cultural officer took me to the village. There was a long line up of people awaiting their gift for their ailments. The cultural officer manned the line. For hours, one stepped up after the other, going away happy. Finally the line ended. Now I was invited further invited into their village. I immediately noticed a very tall stately female around whom many little children gathered. Some clung to her legs and arms. My inner child wished to do the same. After walking around some it came to my awareness that the people were dressed in western clothing rather than their native ones.

Then I saw a small group of males and females gather in their native attire. They had dressed up on my behalf. The men wore a red and blue checkered cloth wrapped around their bodies, somewhat in a similar way as Hindu females wrap their Sarris. The men also had their long poles with them. The females of this small group had donned their beaded necklaces of many layers, in size order. Their necklaces, I recalled was customary for females to begin working on at an early age and continue working on into adulthood. By that time it had reached its full beauty and form.

The small group arrived to express their gratitude for my help. This they proceeded to do by performing their singing and dancing just for me. The men were on one side doing their singing and dancing. Their singing consisted of making sounds like, in a sing/ manner, HHM, HHM, HHM as they, with the help of their long poles jumped high up into the air. The woman stood together close by. They sang along. Those that had their necklaces on bopped their necklaces up and down.

One very beautiful young woman with an extra-ordinary necklace desired to put on my big brimmed hat. In exchange she gave me her necklace to wear. I wanted to join them with the bopping motions. Then I noticed the tall, very regal woman that I had previously admired and longed to be near, showing me, with her shoulders how I could best facilitate the bopping of the necklace up and down. I did my best. Clearly this required much more practice.

For me the celebration and gift ended too quickly. I was leaving their village. I then noticed the regal matriarch, as I realized that, indeed she was, walking at a respectful distance with me, about 5 or 6 feet, on my heart side as I slowly left the village. She walked all along the way, looking at me. Only some tall grasses and the 5-6 feet, separated us. As I reached the edge of the village, I felt a deep and intense sense of loss and grief. I had an intense desire to run over to hug her, tell her I loved her and to call her mother. Then I recalled that in a previous lifetime, in England, she actually was my mother. Quiet tears rolled down my cheeks. Thank you my dear, beloved mother for then and for now.

  Now, one of the many differences between the indigenous people from westerners, especially 'educated' ones is that seeing one example was enough for them to believe and trust. With westerners and 'educated' people, they are too clever for that. Even upon seeing example after example, they disbelieve. Even experiencing the value once they still disbelieve it as unscientific, an illusion, a trick and so forth. This is why I refrained from trying to convince people in the United States that what I have to share has value.

At some point while I was still in Arusha a couple came to see me and requested for me to assist with their little girl. I am unsure and I never asked them how they heard of me or found me. All I know is there they were at the place that I was staying at. They brought their little girl with them. The darling child was as limp as a rag doll. The parents stated that though she was old enough, she was unable to even lift her head, much less hold her bottle to drink. It became clear that they were observant of the christian religion. I requested them to lay their child on a table and requested them to pray, in their own way and I would open myself up as a vessel on behalf of their darling child. We did this together for a while, until I was inner guided to stop.

 I informed them as to when I was leaving the area and going to Zanzibar and where I was going to stay. I invited them, that if they so desired they could come there for more of the same.

The cultural officer who made my visit with the Massai possible, at some point complained to me about an intense headache. I asked him to sit and directed energy towards a part of his head where I was inner guided to. Abruptly he stated that he could see the clock on the wall. I was puzzled. Then he explained that he wore glasses as needed and without his glasses he was unable to see the clock. So here it was, in addition to his headache having left, his vision also got healed. I kept in contact with him on the telephone while I was in Tanzania. Each time he reported that his glasses were still in the drawer where he kept them, without any need to use them.

At another point of me still being in Arusha, this same cultural office brought over a young man to where I was staying. The young man had also accepted christianity. They explained that since the age of five the young mans' vision bit by bit decreased to the present time that he was unable to even see his own hands in front of his face. I was directed to focus energy to part of his head.

Then, honoring his path, I gave him instructions to make a list of any and all ways that he has felt he was hurt by others and how he said or did things that harmed others. I asked him to 'repent' for his causing others grief and pain and to release the others from any animosity that he could still be feeling towards them for their ill treatment of him. Further, that after that was done to take a bath keeping in mind that with the water he is cleansing and purifying himself and is being renewed. Lastly I told him to return the next day after all the instructions was completed.

Sure enough he arrived with his escort. Again I was inner guided to focus the energy towards his head. When that felt complete, the young man walked out into the street. He returned beaming with a wide smile. He could see up and down the street. Perfect vision. I was much overwhelmed, even, in some way more so than with the little infant with the cerebral malaria. I am unsure why. I felt very humbled and felt like falling to my knees. As this would have been contrary to my belief system, I just focused on my intense feeling of being overwhelmed, humbled and wanting to cry.

It was now towards the end of my stay in Arusha.it suddenly came to me that I was so close to the Ngorongoro National Park and remembered my wonderful gift from the lion being while I was meditating before my journey. I contacted someone who took people out on safari. He offered a trip either at dawn or dusk. I told him of my request, to see lions. Dawn, he stated would probably be most optimum.

 Dawn it was and off we went. I and he were alone together. I had my tiny binoculars along. We rode and rode, got stuck in mud, however the desired lion remained unseen. Then he stated to me that he often takes people out on safari, even for a complete week and never see lions.

Antelopes and many other animals roam about freely so they are easy to see, however seeing lions is a rare occurrence. I refused to fully accept his discouraging words. I tried to reassure myself by saying to myself: the lion had come to me in my meditation and came thru the Muslim medicine woman, surely it would gift me with seeing him.

Suddenly, the driver stopped the van and stated, look over there, pointing. My hands shook and I lifted my binoculars to my eyes, however I was unable to see them. He handed me his big binoculars, I focused and finally saw them.

There was the male with his big mane, his female mate and a younger male, their offspring huddled together. I began to cry as I heard him say to me: 'See, **I have brought out my family for you to see**'. Tears kept on rolling downs my face. Gratitude, gratitude my dear, dear lions.

We drove on towards leaving the park. On our way out we passed two other safari vans. Neither of them had seen the lions. Only I got to see the lions that day in the Ngorongoro national park. It was my last day in

Arusha. The next day I took an airplane to Zanzibar to stay for a few days by the sea, to rest up.

The place I stayed at was lovely, I had a small cabin all to myself, overlooking the ocean. Very peaceful. I really needed it. The trip, so far has been very intense on many levels and tiring.

 The first morning I went for a walk on the beach. I noticed a man fixing his boat with what appeared like a tarlike concoction. I surmised he was a fisherman. I sat and watched him at his task of repairing. We stayed in silence, together, with neither of us being able to speak the others verbal language. However there is a communication that can happen without words. I felt this with him.

The next morning I again went to visit and to watch him fix his boat. This time he had his little boy, around the age of two or three with him. He held his son and pointed to his sons puffed up lips. Something either bit him, or perhaps he fell down and got hurt. In either case the lips were inflamed and it appeared it had been like that for quite a while. I directed energy to the child's lips.

The next day, I returned to the place. Here he was again with his son and again he pointed to his sons lip. And there it was, all healed and well.

Now how in the world did this man intuit that I could somehow help his sons lip? Interesting. There are those that recognize others in a way that the masses are unable to recognize, much less appreciate. This fisherman was truly connected. He felt to me as if he was my brother. On a deep level, he was. As I returned to my cabin I found, right outside my door, a bunch of the most beautiful sea shells I had ever seen. They were all cleaned up, gleaming and shining. Clearly a gift from the fisherman for his sons healing. Words would only have gotten in the way.

Then the couple with their little girl showed up. They had traveled far to get to Zanzibar. Please recall that I took an airplane to get from Arusha to Zanzibar. They took a boat, probably it was more affordable.

They reported that their beloved daughter had made great improvements, picking up her own head and neck and even holding her own bottle. So, we proceeded to do the same as we did back in Arusha. I again shared that from Zanzibar I was going to Dar Es Salaam and where I was going to stay, also indicating that I was going to fly back to the States on the following day, therefore there was only a small window when they could find me.

 Sure enough, they showed up again, smiling that, yet again their beloved child had made headway. We did our routine and before parting I told them that I will continue sending energy whenever I was inner guided to do so and told them to feel free to connect through the ethers as I will hear them calling to me. This, I did until I was inner guided to stop.

 Many years later I was informed that the little girl was grown, got married, gave birth to four children and only needed to use crutches once in a while. Hip hip hurrah!

At some point, I am unable to recall the exact order of my journeys here and there, I was led to go to Texas. There I connected the Buddhist community and visited with a Tibetan Lama. I am without memory of how it unfolded or came about, however, I very clearly recall sitting across from him at his table. I also very distinctly recall how at some point he smiled, giggled in a childlike manner and stated that I had 'Compassion Power'. He requested to be a recipient. I gladly obliged.

On another journey, this one to Morocco, I was invited to stay for a weekend with a family. Upon arrival at their home, their teen age son happened to mention that a tooth of his was hurting him. Upon becoming free from that pain, he ran into his home and told his parents what had occurred.

 His father then told me that he has had a severe pain in his wrist. I was clearly inner guided that I needed to let it be. I told him so. I was also guided to tell him, and I did, that he first has to deal with the root of why the pain was there. This he adamantly refused to do and proceeded to demand that I do it anyway. On his third insistence, I did as he requested. By the morning his pain had increased. He complained to me, upon which I retorted that I had clearly told him that I had to let it be and he had to deal with why the pain was there in the first place. Due to his insistence, he got his answer by the pain having increased.

This was also a good lesson for me, that regardless of the others insistence, when I am inner guided to let it be, for me to do so.

Interestingly, this same man took me to some important politicians home to visit. The politician upon being told of what can happen through me asked me to do something to help his son. I was directed to sit outside his sons closed door and do what I could. As I sat there, I became quite ill. This very yuckee energy seeped out from the sons' room into me. I became increasingly concerned for my safety and welfare. I went outside and sat down on the earth in hopes of getting well again. That took quite a while due to the immense toxicity that had invaded me from the young man, that I was informed was due his use of drugs and his violent behaviors.

Another lesson for me. I, eventually developed a protocol for myself. This was as follows. Upon being requested to support another with this or that, I began with asking my inner guidance: is it for the others highest good to receive the benefit of what comes through me? Do I have permission to assist? To do it now? Is it on me to assist? Will it benefit the other? I further asked whatever else I needed to hear, and ask to make sure that all the basis were covered.

 I also became aware that often it was too early to help and if I did so too early then the other would develop another dis-ease to give them the opportunity to yet again deal with the root of why the discomfort occurred in the first place.

There is a reason and opportunity to learn and make changes in ourselves as needed for our benefit and to benefit all that is. As we grow, all the cosmos benefits. So, in effect when I am overly 'helpful' it can, indeed harm the other by them having to begin all over again to learn what is the root of the matter.

I wonder as I write this why I have avoided asking for insight regarding my safety. Is it my tendency to regard myself as less important than the other? Is it my natural inclination to help others, regardless of what happens to me? Is there a self-sacrifice thread from many lives of doing that?

I am aware that, especially clearing yuckee energy can, and often is very dangerous. One has to be very grounded, have a strong boundary/shield around oneself and know when one has reached ones limit and stop before it is too late. Then there is also the situation that one has to proceed regardless of the danger to oneself. Some things just need to me done. And when getting clear guidance to proceed then so. I had this happen on one or two occasions, however, this incident in Morocco was NOT one of those. I neither asked nor was I told to refrain.

Another growth opportunity for me. May I remember for the next time.

Upon getting all this knowledge and awareness I wondered why, in Tanzania the rate of 'success' was so high? Also with the few that came to me as clients at the company I worked for as a psychotherapist.

What came to me was that those that came to me both at work and in Tanzania had already reached their level of having dealt with the root of the matter, unbeknown to them. All systems, had, thereby indicated GO for them to receive and gain by it. The complete process of being a vessel, in this life, was new to me and the cosmos chose to have me 'succeed' as a base level, to know that this 'works'.

Then it was time for me to grow and be aware of the other side to gain discernment, clarity that often the systems are unready for GO. Often others and I are eager to fix it, have unpleasantness be gone. However, often we are still without readiness. More inner work and awareness needs to occur to make sure that what caused the dis-ease in the first place had been taken care of. If the client is unaware, then I, the facilitator needs to listen and hear whether the systems are indeed GO both for the client and for myself, and with them, and is it now? Many variables. Cover all the bases.

I also found that in places where the other and I were without a common speaking language, it was easier and clearer. It was either yes of no. However in places where there was a common speaking language then more often I was told yes, however it needs to be postponed until the client deals with this or that, the root of why the ailment was there in the first place. Therefore in these incidents, both my psychotherapist and energy worker hats were utilized if the client was open to it.

Most of us opt for a quick fix. That is one reason the masses opt to go to the medical field, to get a quick fix, a drug, have surgery, anything to avoid dealing with the 'why it all occurred in the first place'.

To better clarify, when our system first goes out of kilter, it first occurs in our spiritual body. If ignored then it also occurs in our mental body and then progresses into our emotional body. By this time it already has affected us in three of our four bodies. Then, finally it effects our physical body in addition to the other three.

This is the stage where the masses typically go for help to the medical field. The medical field then deals only with the physical body. The masses consider the physical body the most important. The masses are most likely to be caring and concerned for other people when they have a physical body dis-ease. The physical body is our heaviest and lowest form of energy and vibratory frequency. People have it all backwards.

The most important time to take immediate action is when our spirit body gets out of harmony. If one is unaware of what that feels like or is about, or even care, then our system ups the ante and we get a more intense sign, our mental and emotional bodies. At that time it becomes very evident that there is definitely something off in our life. We get many clues and clear evidence in many parts of our lives. Unfortunately, emotional and mental challenges have been judged harshly, it has been denied as it being all made up all in the others mind. It is judged that it was their own doing, the ailing one feels shamed and humiliated as they are called 'crazy', 'a lunatic' or another demeaning term. People with ailments in the emotional and mental bodies are often locked up, drugged into oblivion and severely abused. Of course all this kind of treatment only exacerbates the situation. Then when physical ailments arise, there is often a gladness that comes to the ailing one, oh, yes, now they will be validated that they actually have a legitimate dis-ease. Again, getting it all backwards.

Returning a bit to Morocco. I connected with another religious community and explained what comes through me. Suddenly I was inundated with requests, which on its own would have been fine. However, there was an element that scared me to my core. I felt I was being worshipped and treated as if I was an idol. That is the easiest way to loose ones path. In the Jewish tradition there is a warning to flee from honor. This I did in Morocco away from the community that felt to me as if they were doing idol worship. It was clear to me how quickly one can totally lose ones way and with it undo years, or lifetimes of work of focusing on elevating oneself to a purer level of beingness. One minute one can be humble and the next minute it can all be lost.

Next there was Brazil. I actually went there for some special healing available in only two countries in the world. The place it resonated better with me was Brazil. I was, gratefully, fortunate to find a couple of people who this unique technique who had the integrity to support me in a beneficial way. On this journey, yet again after two police officers helped me make some beneficial contacts I felt inner guided to offer, as reciprocity, to support them in a beneficial way for them. They both accepted and received their advancement in their journey in life. I believe it is important to have harmony in receiving and giving wherever and however is most appropriate.

Then on to Israel. A couple found their way to me or me to them. There we were, together. I was invited to the land upon which they lived. There I was drawn to a site that I was informed was an ancient Medicine wheel. Medicine wheels exist all over the world. They are called by many different names. The bottom line is the same. It is a sacred circle, optimum for raising oneself to a higher level of awareness. I informed the female and showed her the exact place and how far the wheel extended. I also that she may wish to consider putting down rocks or some other signs to indicate the boundaries of the wheel. In addition, gave her information about medicine wheels.

Then we sat outside, all three of us in a tent in the evening and they shared this and that challenges they had and were having. From the list, the most significant occurrence was that two of their homes were burned down to the ground. That is very intense! I felt guided to say for them to choose which of them, as the family representative, would have a session with me to support a shift out of the families recurring disasters. The husband offered himself.

The next day he and I met at his home. We sat together for hours to really deal with the core issues. His energy kept shifting and shifting into being more and more cleared. At one point he actually threw up some yuck. Fortunately, a bit earlier I was inner guided to prepare a pail, just in case. At some point, the husband and I had had maxed out the session for him.

Next was Singapore where I was led to connect with the Sikh community. It was a lovely connection for all of us. To stay on focus I will just fast forward to an incident where a unique experience took place. The youth group of the Sikh temple I went to invited me to be a guest and go with them to a retreat in the outskirts of the city limits. I joined, gratefully.

On the way over to the camping place I noticed a small pond like area. While at the camp grounds I invited several of the group to go with me there. Several of them brought along their drums. I was inner guided to take along a clear crystal I had in my bag. We stood along the banks of the pond like place. Parts had tall plants growing out of the water.

We started chanting and the two who brought their drums along, invited their drums to sing. Beforehand, I had handed the crystal to one men and told him to throw the crystal into the water when I tell him to. The chanting and drumming build up to a crescendo. Suddenly the yell came out of me, 'Throw It Now' and I fell backwards. My fall was blocked by one of the drums, scraping my skin badly. However, it did prevent me from falling completely and perhaps being more injured. I looked at and into the water, I saw and felt a great shift in its energy, I saw light beings, that some would call angels floating here and there in a beneficial and loving way. It was an amazing scene! As far as I know, I was the only one who saw. However, most present felt a beneficial shift.

I was made aware that this was a most valuable and important shift that needed to be made. It benefited way past the boundaries of what appeared to be just a small pond. Indeed, I had been informed while we were on the way to the camp and passed the water that it was on us to support the much needed shift that it was ready for. We did it, yeah us! This group of young Sikhs were very aware and had wonderful, pure energy. I extend gratitude to them. Also gratitude for the information and all the light beings who made it all possible. Ik Ongkar. Pure manifestation.

At this juncture I would like to further explain. With the first stories of peoples 'getting well' while I was working as a psychotherapist I was living in Baltimore, Maryland. Baltimore is a big city, with multicultures, and multireligions living together. Therefore, there was a greater tendency towards people being open to a 'different' idea and way of doing something. Then I was inner guided to move to Southwest Virginia to create a Spiritual healing center and with it have holistic practitioners assist and support others in their own healing. It is the idea of 'doing with' versus 'doing for' or 'doing to'. Generally speaking, holistic practitioners have more of a tendency towards 'empowering' their clients versus dominating them, which is what, generally speaking the medical field tends to do. In addition, the plan was also to introduce meditation and, perhaps most importantly invite people of all belief systems, all races and paths to come and sit together in a circle of peace. The center never happened as I understood that it was meant to be. The people of the area were closed to all I had to offer. I had a neighbor tell me that if the center would have taken off, the neighbors would have burned my home down.

Therefore, upon my return to Virginia from one of my glorious trips here and there a wisdom came to me. Do it differently. I listened up. This new way was that whomever I spoke to be it on the telephone or face to face, for me to be a pure vessel similarly as to when the other requests my support. This meant even something 'outlandish' like: I am in Walmart, a huge store that offers fresh produce, technical supplies, hardware, household items, clothing, and on and on. Very popular for the masses. So let's say there I am in Walmart doing my own shopping. Suddenly I am inner guided to go to another aisle as someone there needs to be told something. So I head on over there. There I am guided to go near a specific customer. I saunter over there as if I am looking for an item near where she is standing. I then, casually, ask them something about an item on one of the shelves. She replies. Then, softly and gently the 'words the other needed to hear' comes forth. That is it. I had done what I was led to do.

I am confident that many, consciously, totally disregarded, what was said through me. And, I am also aware that a seed had been planted. Maybe they did hear it in moment and it stayed with them. Or perhaps in the moment they just carried on and forgot the words totally. However, later on, at some point be it later that day, month or year, or even many years later those words came back to them. Maybe an incident reminded them. Maybe something someone else said that reminded them. At some point they were able to fully benefit from what came thru me to tell them on that faithful moment in Walmart.

From then on, that is how the vessel hood came through from me. There were many potential benefits. One, if the words that came out were more in the alignment with what a psychotherapist would say it gave an opportunity for the other to benefit as if they went for a session, something that the masses, typically avoid doing. This could be due to monetary restraints or ideology ones.

If the words that came through me was more inclined to be stated by someone like me, a spiritual being, someone who desired to sit in a circle of peace like in the 'great vision' of Black Elk, leader of the Lakota native American path. In his 'great vision' he saw the 'Hoop of all the nations' sitting in a circle of peace. That was and is my great vision also. In that instance, the chance of someone seeking me out were pretty slim to none. However, regardless of where or when I was, and I casually walked over and uttered a few words and then moved on, there it was. They got the message.

In time this method got and still gets to be utilized constantly in every phone call, with every meeting, with every opportunity. This applied to when people came to the home I lived in to fix this or that. This was the constant mode. Being a vessel constantly with what words came through me, what feelings were exhibited through me and what actions.

There was, for me, the challenge of differentiating between what was for them and what was for me. Eventually it became clear to me that my need was their need and their needs were my need. We are one, what truly benefits one of us benefits all of us. Instead of feeling like I was becoming a puppet, I understood, accepted and was/am grateful to be as pure a vessel as possible to support others in their lives much more than if I hung up a sign to indicate 'psychotherapist' or any other title. Basic bottom line, monetarily, it was free.

Beyond that the masses tend only to seek out support from those others they are accustomed to: medical doctors, lawyers and such. Their mimic their own communities' norms. This is similar in many parts of the world. I have lived and continue to be what many would call, 'counter-culture'. I live more and more 'out of the box' with progressive and liberal ideas. My intention has been to, eventually, be totally free of all boxes. Boxes are prisons. Boxes limit consciousness and ways of being. I am a strong component of 'expanded consciousness'. Moving Beyond. Always moving beyond.

So there it is. Everyone who has any contact with me has the good fortune to be presented with options to choose from, whereas before our 'meeting' there was none.

Some areas in this country of the United States, like in the big cities, people have a tendency to be more open and receptive of something new and different than they grew up with, due to their constant interaction with multicultural populations' surrounding them constantly. With it they expand, experiment, walk a new path.

However, I have found that in small cities and towns, the masses are more closed, or totally closed to everything else besides what has been since the 'cave beings', so to speak. Total limiting consciousness.

Of course there is the great value of many indigenous and aboriginal ways of being. However what is hereby being referred to is totally different than that. These populations who embody what I call 'limited consciousness' has nothing to do with indigenous/aboriginal wisdoms and ways. Indeed, totally the opposite. I have found great richness and value in being around and with many indigenous and aboriginal peoples. However, what I am referring to is 'small town' mentality that had formed and stayed stuck in that mode forever.

Hopefully, you, the readers of this book, will hear these words and accept it with the intention that it is intended. Being closed to anything 'new', being 'ultra conservative', passing on from generation to generation the same limited consciousness have kept many 'small town' peoples stuck in 'small town mentality and ways of thinking' and with it causing great harm to all involved directly and indirectly. We either 'evolve' or we 'devolve'. Very sadly, worldwide, the masses have chosen to 'devolve', self-destruct and with it take the world down with them.

We, as people, are destroying our homeland, mother earth and ourselves. We either wake up or act very quickly or we will cease to exist, as we now know it. Many of us are tenaciously holding on to old harmful patterns as if our lives depended on it. It is just the opposite, my dear readers, just the opposite.

 It is vital for us to be able to differentiate and discern what is most beneficial for us to hold on to and what we absolutely must let go of, and do it now. To do this is a must for the future generations, our children, grandchildren and further down the line. It is our duty and obligation!

'Arise, awaken and remember'!

In a third world country like Tanzania, where the indigenous, christian and Muslim medicine woman and men often blended together more than one path. With it the multitudes also embodied the very rich culture of their ancestors' wisdoms of native indigenous/aboriginal mindset. There was also, with it, a childlike openness to trying and then easily accepting 'new' into their lives.

As stated earlier, with the Massai, one example of a man saying 'show me' and he immediately got well was enough for his village people to line up to receive the benefit of a brand new way that they had never before heard of. The multitudes 'childlike openness' was most refreshing and freeing for both them and me.

Then there was the trip to Greece. Before leaving I flipped through a travel guide, and I specifically remember, on the left side of the page there was at the top a boxed in area. In it was written about a place called Kalavrita where, during World War II the Nazis slaughtered every male over the age of 13. I was horrified and intended to refrain from going there.

At some point in my journey, I was on one of the islands in a big city and I longed to be in a peaceful, quiet area. I stopped a police officer and asked him if he could recommend such a place for me. Without even thinking he stated Kalavrita. I had, by that time totally forgotten that that place was the one I was determined to avoid. So I went to Kalavrita.

Once I arrived, I went to services at the Greek Orthodox Church. I, typically, visit houses of worship, whichever religion when I go hither and yon, going with respect and honoring in my heart. So there I am in the women's section, dressed appropriately as is their custom. My attention was drawn towards this elderly female sitting against the wall, she was in full view as her chair was turned so that she faced out towards the rest of the congregation. Something pulled me towards looking at her again and again.

After services I seeked out the cultural officer building. I asked about the elder woman. Immediately they knew who I was talking about due to my description. She related the horror story that I had read about way back while flipping through the travel guide. The cultural officer explained that this self-same woman had every male family member slaughtered by the Nazis on that day. She was the only one of two people that were still alive now, and present when the massacre occurred.

So, there I was after all. I understood that I was meant to go there and 'DO what needed to be done'. I got directions on where the spot was and walked there. It was easy to find the spot due to, beside the directions, the energy of the place pulled me to it.

 I entered the hill and was inner guided to go to a far side of the area where I had the complete area in my full line of vision. I focused and opened myself up, as usual, to be a pure and clear vessel to assist and support what is for the benefit of all.

Different tunes emerged from the depths of my beingness, one tune after another without rhyme or reason that I could understand as to why this tune or that one either sung our loud or hummed out loud. I was a vessel and welcomed it to flow through.

As this singing continued, I began seeing souls starting to float up and up. Some went by themselves, some in a group. First it was just here and there, then more and more souls rose up from the ground and floated up and up. I started to get choked up from emotions. However, I continued the tunes as it came to me. At some point the flow of tunes stopped. I still observed some souls floating up, and then it all stopped. Some souls may have decided to stay on. That was their choice.

My commitment was to be a vessel and refrain from any imposing that I may have wished or desired. The souls, like us in the physical form have a right of self-determination. When we intrude interfere or impose our will it is akin to abusing the other. Furthermore it is arrogant for any of us to assume that we know best what the other 'needs' to do, or as to what is really, in the bigger picture, the best at this time in this place. We must avoid any chance that we may, indeed, be creating more harm and hardship for the other.

I left the area, quiet overwhelmed and went for a long walk in the mountains to take it all in and return to earth. Soon thereafter, I was guided to leave Kalavrita.

Another incidence occurred in another part of Greece, on another island. I again had just gone to another service at the Greek Orthodox Church. I love hearing the Greek language, and especially in prayer, the tunes and rhythm I find very healing.

Anyway, as I left I found myself walking into a store that had various crystals in the window. Inside there was the owner, a female. We sat and talked for a bit and at some point she shared that she was without children, however she was pregnant once however she started bleeding and there was no more pregnancy. She stated this was many years ago and she was still grieving and unable to put it to rest.

I quieted myself and listened. Sure enough words flowed out from me. The woman was told that the soul of the fetus wished to express her gratitude for the woman allowing herself to be a vessel for her, the fetuses' soul, to clear some parts of her soul that needed repair. With her potential mothers allowing herself to be a vessel to grant the opportunity for her, the fetuses' soul to fix and repair what needed to be freed, granting her soul to go to a higher level. The soul again expressed gratitude to her potential mother and wished her well. That was it.

I looked up and saw the woman had tears streaming down her face. We were both silent for a while. Thereafter, the woman expressed her gratitude and that she now felt consoled and comforted. There was a purpose after all, she had a child whom she helped to grow, evolve and the child even expressed gratitude and wished her well. Many mothers who toil for years raising a child never get that. I bid the woman all the best and left her store.

Another journey led me to Papua New Guinea and, with it, Indonesia. Two pieces of information appeared to be the catalysts for this journey.

The first was the longing I had to experience being in a matriarchal society. We all have been indoctrinated and living in a very dogmatic Patriarchy, now for over 7,000 years, or longer. Male and masculine consciousness probably existed from the beginning of time perhaps due to men being, typically, stronger, physically, than females. This was and continuous to be a disparity. Power over females. However, about 7,000 years ago this pattern shifted into a much higher gear with the invention of 'a male deity in the sky'. Since then, both male and masculine consciousness took over, to all of our detriment.

What is masculine versus feminine consciousness? Masculine consciousness, residing in the left side of our brains, includes: power and control over, aggression, domination, win-lose mentality and the like. Feminine mentality includes: peace, compromise, win-win mentality, spirituality, creativity and the like. Feminine consciousness on the right side of our brain. You may wonder why two such differences?

In a 'good enough' healthy individual, the two sides of our brains are in harmony and we utilize the most optimum action for each situation. Yes setting limits with others who are harming us is vital for our survival. This, whether we do it verbally by saying, 'no, get away' or leaving a destructive relationship. The power to say "NO" and really mean it comes from our masculine side. Allowing ourselves to be abused is in alignment with our feminine side. This is just one tiny example how and why we need both options and ways of being depending on the situation. Unfortunately, very few of us are in harmony with one side complimenting the other. We are mostly lopsided. It takes wisdom and a commitment to do our best to bring the two sides of our brains, and with it our complete ways of thinking and be-ing, to shift it all into being healthier and well rounded. I wish us all success in achieving this.

This was, what I thought the reason to go to Indonesia, to experience a matriarchy. In the world I had been aware that the Native American tribe of the Hopi Indians was such. Then I heard of Bukitingi in Indonesia being another. I desired to visit and experience. I went and visited Bukitingi. Mostly it was disappointing. The set up was the same, only instead of males dominating, it was the females.

I had remembered reading about Old Europe, written by Marija Gimbutas, an archeologist. She identified the areas and people to be more like a matriarchy, however, indeed it was androgynous with both genders being of equal value and worth. There was harmony and accord. There was peace. They were without any weapons and totally free of any aggression whatsoever. Mother earth and all of nature was honored and respected. This existed for thousands of years in that way. Then men from the north arrived on horseback, with weapons and brought the idea of a male deity in the sky who demanded sacrifices of both animals and other people. This began poisonous pedagogy, wars, violence and masculine consciousness domination into our world. From then on, we have gone downhill.

So, here I was in Bukitingi feeling very disappointed. The only thing that was different was who dominated rather than peace and harmony as I envisioned and hoped that it would be.

However, there was a ray of sun gifted me. During my visit with a matriarchal family, the elder female, a grandmother looked me in the eyes and clearly and with power stated: "Always remember to hold your own, with your head held high, shoulder to shoulder with the other." Great wisdom. Indeed, a gift. I, looking back upon this, feel in my beingness that the elder saw and intuited that I greatly needed that. She probably saw my body posture, heard my speaking voice and, gratefully chose to gift me with her stating out loud a remedy to help me come more into my power, to be able to hold my own with others. Thank you elder Bukitingi grandmother.

To date, regrettably, I have yet to achieve that on a consistent basis. This challenge of mine has been with me for long time. Actually, for many lifetimes.

It would have been great to have a grandmother to remind me in my formative years, like that elder Bukitingi grandmother did that day. To have it be told to me in my formative years would have co-created a totally different me, and with it a very different life for me.

I am grateful I was now reminded of the elders' wonderful words. While she was saying this to me she was sitting up straight, with her head held high, shoulders back, her back straight. She was a giant, a powerful force, and yet, towards me clearly caring and loving. She was a great vessel to say exactly what she stated and to declare it with authority and gentleness rolled into one. I was and am grateful.

Then why Papua New Guinea? Well, on the surface, it appeared that it was due to information I read that declared that Papua New Guinea was the only place on Mother Earth where people have actually improved on nature rather than destroying it. That felt and feels vital to me. Yes I absolutely wanted to see and experience that wonderful phenomenon while it still existed.

With all our greed, any day they could also join others worldwide into desecrating and destroying our precious Mother Earth. So off I went.

I arrived at the airport and I had no place to go to stay. I am unsure how if came about, but one of the men at the airport invited me to his home. Now writing this and looking back, I am surprised at my willingness to except such an invitation. I was totally without any fear or apprehension. Gratefully, here I am, writing this. A good sign.

I related to him my desire to be with the Papuan population. I found out that they mostly lived in the mountains, high up. He made arrangements with a family who agreed to welcome me and this young man to set up a little tent and sleep on their tiny property.

The young man took me shopping. I purchased a giant bag of rice to cook for me and to share it with the family. By the end of my stay the gigantic bag was still quiet full. I left all of it, and most of my belongings for the family. My clothes I gave to the two females.

After sleeping with the young man together in the tiny tent I told him he needed to go and send a female in his stead. He had done nothing inappropriate, however he and his energy felt very off for me, especially with the close proximity we were in all night long. He was gone and I was left without a translator for, best I recall, two or three days.

However, I am getting ahead of myself.

 Once all the shopping was done and gathered together, I put on my backpack and he carried his things and all the food. It was a very long and steep walk up the mountain. Best I recall it was about a two hour trek up the mountain, maybe more. We finally arrived.

 Immediately I noticed, right before we reached the homestead of the family we were to stay at, that there was this incredible waterfall, pond combination that began at the height, very near the homestead of the family we were going to stay at, and the water ran down a slope. Children were frolicking, laughing and having an all-around, glorious fun. How fabulous.

When we arrived I met with the husband and wife, the wifes' mother and their teen-age son. They had this tiny homestead which included their small hut that the husband had built out of twigs, leaves, straw and pieces of scrap wood he must have found somewhere. Right behind their hut was a hole. This was the bathroom. Then there was the barn for their pigs. In the center were some benches to sit on.

That is where I cooked my food the traditional way by building a fire and so forth. After all, the rice had to be cooked. For their meals, they dug a hole in the ground, put on some hot stones and rocks that they first heated up the way I cooked my rice. They put some of the heated rocks on the bottom, piled in their meal to be and then piled over them more heated rocks. That cooked and cooked what seemed to me like forever. Mostly all I ever saw them eat was sweet potato and sometimes the greens that grew with the sweet potatoes.

The families' schedule was as follows. The husband, while I was there always stayed by the homestead. His job was to make sure that the hut they lived in was intact and made whatever repairs needed to be done regularly. His other job was to discuss with the men of the community 'important matters'. While I was there, that was his daily routine. I am unable to know whether that was his regular routine or did he stay put all day to keep me company? The son disappeared in the early morning and returned at night to have supper and go to sleep with his family. All four of them slept together in the small hut.

The two females also left early in the morning to tend to their garden where they planted and grew the sweet potatoes for their meals. The only tool they had and took with them was a stick, one for each of them. I was unaware of how far or where their garden was or what kind of a setup it was. Was it a community garden in which each family had their own plot?

I refrained from asking any questions, being unaware of how it would be received and perceived. All day the women were gone. They returned in time to cook the evening meal, eat, we all sat by the fire a bit, the husband played his tiny instrument that he made and played the same song. Always the same song. It was sweet and gentle.

The wifes' clothing consisted of a fabric skirt and that was all. The grandmothers, best I recall, was the same. Many of the other females that I saw only had a skirt made out of hay, similar to what I have seen females of Hawaii wear. The men that I saw mostly just wore a gourd over their private part, and to hold up the gourd they had a rope or string tied to the gourd and to their waist to give the gourd height. However, the husband and son wore loose swim shorts made of cloth. I was grateful for that. It appeared, the best I could tell that the missionaries had some effect on them.

The grandmother and wife, for all practical purposes, had little or nothing to do with me. Only on one occasion after the Indonesian male got replaced by an Indonesian family did the grandmother make some hand motions during the meal. I was puzzled, what did her hand signals mean? The girl translated for me: "An Angel Came Down From Heaven To Us", referring to me. I was very surprised and grateful.

I was surprised because she never acknowledged in any way my presence. I felt with her and her daughter that I was invisible. Maybe it was a cultural thing? At some point the husband stated that he will: "Build A Hotel And Name It After Me To Attract Others Like Me."

Looking back, I now recall, I never heard any of them talk to each other, and certainly NEVER any raised voices. If they talked in my presence it must have been very soft and quiet.

Mostly I remember that when, during the day men came to visit the husband, they did talk, however, that was also very soft and quiet. Maybe the culture in general, or maybe the custom was to talk softer when others were about? Questions, so many questions I refrained from asking, lest I would be intruding or being out of line in their culture. Best to be cautious, respectful and honoring.

Before I left I gave the two women a cotton skirt, and under pants. Besides sundries and this and that, I left the gigantic bag of rice for them. Best I recall it was either a 25 or 50 pound bag it was enormous and very heavy. It was the biggest bag of rice that the store had. I bought the biggest size to make sure that there would be plenty left over for the family I stayed with. Reciprocity is important.

For my last night there I told the family to invite their neighbors for a meal. We cooked a lot of rice. The husband played his tune.

The husband had this incredible habit. He was at all times very respectful of my space. I felt his gentle heart and spirit, and, clearly he cared for me in a respectful way. The first time he did what I am about to relate I was surprised and taken aback. He reached over wrapped his two hands around a spot on my arm above my wrist and below my elbow, typically on my right arm due to his siting on that side of me. Then he gently squeezed and made m- m-m sounds. I understood that this was his very respectful way of hugging me. **He did this regularly, endearment, so sweet and innocent.**

Backtracking a bit: After the Indonesian male left to send a female in his stead I was without a translator for two days. That was fine. I felt safe with the husband being my guardian. On the first day I went out for a walk. It was glorious. All of nature had definitely been improved on. Places where the soil was in danger due to water runoff, was mindfully built up with natures best. The air smelled clean and pure. I invited into me the pristine air and environment.

I was walking along, enjoying myself when suddenly I found myself being surrounded by three tiny boys, about ages six or seven. I gathered that the husband was worried about me and sent the boys to make sure I was ok and to make sure I found my way back. The boys laughed and jumped around me. I was inner guided to initiate them and pass on the baton to them the ability to be able to support their community with the healing for others as needed. This was to occur when they got older. Basically they got initiated for what was to occur in the future. I always mindfully ask as to where and when the baton needed to be passed on so there would be someone else to take my place and be available for their people.

The process with the three tiny boys went like this: I stated to each one in turn, pointing to them 'Doctor" taped them on their shoulder as if I was knighting them and then shook their hand. I repeated that routine with each. All three of us then proceeded to head back. All three smiled widely and happily as if they understood. Who knows? I did what I was guided to. That is all I could do.

Before I left I was also inner guided to initiate the son. This was more subtle and without any physical contact. I had brought an eagle feather with me. This I gave to him and he understood. The first time I tried he refused. Later, I understood I had made the error of doing in in front of others. Later I waited for us to be alone and offered the feather again. Then he accepted it. Now I had good confirmation that I had heard inner guidance well to offer it to him as I saw that he was, indeed, very aware of the wisdom of refusing it in front of others and only accepted it when we were alone. He was way ahead of me already. He knew that he was safer without others knowing about receiving powers. That was ancient wisdom from his ancestors. Awesome!

Then it was time for the girl and I to leave. The couple and son walked us the complete way down the hill, first I was very surprised, such a long way down just to accompany me in their bare feet? But then I realized upon them also getting on the bus I was getting on that they had coordinated their need to go into town with my leaving. As we arrived in town, we all got off the van.

The wife hugged me goodbye. She told her son to also hug me. He shyly refused. I insisted that it was ok and said goodbye to him. Her son, probably about age 17, was too old to be hugging a woman who was other than close family. He may have never touched a female since his puberty?

The husband began to cry and cried as he did his usual m-m-m-m hug, took longer than usual. I, myself felt like I was saying goodbye to an old friend or brother. Loss and grief overwhelmed me. I was never even told any of their names.

I grieved knowing that I will never see the husband again, never receive his special hug again, and mostly never, ever will I ever have a male both treat me with such caring, concern, love and treat me in a way that I felt completely safe, respected both as me as a hu-being and me as a female.

For me, this was a most special experience! I thought that the main reason I went to Papua was to see and be with the 'only place in Mother Earth that we, people actually improved on nature instead of destroying it'. Yes, there was that. And, yes, that, by itself would have been enough. However, my stay with the Papuan family was much more than that.

They, total strangers, in the scheme of things welcomed me. I was and felt safe. On some deep level they were my family that I never had and wished I did.

Papua, when I was there was one of the very few places in the world that was free of 'modern' There were neither electricity, telephones, nor any other gadgets. Just like Mother Earth intended. There were neither cars nor even bicycles, no radios with batteries, nothing except nature and the people. Fabulous.

The only other place where I found similar were some areas in Tanzania. However, I never stayed overnight by anyone who actually lived like that. I was just never invited. Some the medicine be-ings lived like that however I was only visiting them for a few hours.

This was the first occasion that I recall actually staying overnight, best I recall it was five days altogether in this noise free, quiet peaceful, clean energy magnificent place. I loved it. I wish I could live like that.

 There is so much noise everywhere. When the power goes out in my home my complete bodies relaxes and it says Ahh, yes, quiet at last. I enjoy every minute when that occurs.

 In Papua, in the total silence, my complete mind/body/spirit experienced a flexibility never before felt due to all my bodies being able to relax. In noise, I realize my muscles, nerves and all parts of me tightens up and even contorts in efforts of self-protection.

Regarding Papua, it was a great honor to be there. I am most grateful.

It was this gentle kind male, the husband in Papua, in making the comment to me about 'building a hotel in my name to welcome others like me' brought to my attention and awareness that indeed wherever I go out of this country, the United states I am, and have been a goodwill ambassador. I am unsure how aware most Americans are at how much animosity there is in most countries regarding them. This is due, on one level of how Americans generally behave towards the people of the country they are visiting. Americans typically are arrogant, loud, rude, expecting the residents to speak English. They are demanding and, in general disrespectful. Americans, generally speaking, feel and act like they own the world.

I, on the other hand, constantly remember that I am a guest in the country I am visiting. I immediately learn, know and repeat the word 'thank you' in their language. I believe the words thank you are the most important words in the world. I take with me a dictionary, learn as much as I can before I go and while I am in a country. I respect their customs, traditions and ways of being. I ask questions to best honor their path. Where certain clothing is worn by the women, like with the Muslim women, for example. I dress accordingly. I do my best to be part of, to blend in, and to continue being welcomed and with it enjoy each other's company. I refrain from staying in the tourist areas, and stay away from tourist hotels. I go to live with the people, often away from the cities, to best maximize constant interaction with the people of their country. I remain humble remembering constantly that I am a guest in their homeland. There it is, that is why the darling male in Papua New Guinea stated that he will build a hotel in my name to welcome others like me to come to visit. I never thought of myself as a 'goodwill ambassador' till now. Now I realize, that, indeed I am.

May we all be that, wherever we are and whomever we are with. When I treat others with honor and respect, I am also honoring and respecting myself and what I stand for.

Some or maybe even many readers may wonder, does one have to believe that the 'Compassion Power" will work to have it work. That, my dears is the million dollar question. It depends on when people say they 'believe or that they have faith'. Which aspect are they referring to? Well, most are referring to their 'conscious' mind, which is the part they are more, or only aware of.

 Many people are clueless as what the term the sub-conscious or unconscious really means, and its power or significance. Our conscious mind is our rational mind. It is the place where information and knowledge is stored, from birth about matters we were taught by our parents, teachers and religious leaders. In our conscious mind we have stored the information, clear and simple. Also in our conscious mind are all the indoctrinations we received by those significant others, especially from our first five years of our lives.

At that stage, if there was a specific religion the family followed, very early on it was drummed into us to have faith and belief of the deity being there for us, keeping us safe, the deity knows what is for our best more than we know.

 We are further indoctrinated that parents, like the deity knows what is best for us and that everything they say and do is perfect. By age five most children have been 'well trained' to trust, have faith, follow the rules, accept all that the parents and the deity inflict upon us and to just express gratitude regardless of how and what.

Then there is our subconscious. That is way beyond logic and reason. Our subconscious carries deep seated memories of what was since the beginning of time and first coming to earth as a hu-beings. Every cell of our physical body carries in them all that has ever happened to us, our soul, and for those who are really in touch, can even get in contact with much more. So, in our sub-conscious we are aware of who we really are, free from logic, free from reason.

We are spiritual beings with a deep awareness of all that was and is. It is where our creativity comes from. It is free from the indoctrinations and the limited conscious thinking, patterns and choices that we typically make. When we become aware of sub-conscious and enlist its aid, we truly find out what is really our belief system.

Do we really have faith, belief and trust in our parents, teachers, religious leaders, politicians or are we just repeated it so many times that we have convinced ourselves that 'we believe'. It is only once we remember and reunite ourselves with our sub-conscious and give it the front row seat that we truly find out our real beliefs, values and faith in what and whom. I am referring now, to our deep core, versus what we have been force fed by others. With that renewed connection to our true selves our complete world view shifts

So then we return to your question is it necessary to have faith, trust and belief that the energy I am talking about will work, proving that science is lacking this awareness.

Therefore, if you are talking about your conscious mind, I can only say that it gives us misinformation as we are just repeating what we have been told a million times, so as a rote we just say those words and repeat it over and over again. If you are referring to our sub-conscious I will boldly reply that our sub- conscious has in it the real truth and nothing but the truth. It truly knows, instinctively who is trustworthy and whom to keep away from, if can tell us what is true and what is the opposite.

How to gain the benefit from both, and each in the most beneficial way for our safety and welfare?

If you are truly in touch with your sub-conscious and it clearly indicates to you when someone like me offers what comes through me, you will know, beyond a reasonable doubt. You will relax and be a recipient and benefit.

What about babies and children. Most of them, unawares are still in contact with their sub-conscious. Unaware and free of their conscious minds possibility of interfering.

My beloved readers, depending on where we are in our souls journey depends on how much effort we need to put into doing just that.

May we all succeed speedily in our time.

Love you all, peace be with you and all that is.